Optimizing Her Fertility

A Comprehensive Guide to Enhance Conception through Healthy Diet, Physical Therapy and Fertility Supplements

Winnie R. Adams

Copyright

© 2024 by Winnie R.Adams

Disclaimer:

This book's contents are provided solely for informational reasons. It is not meant to serve as a replacement for expert medical advice, diagnosis, or care. When in doubt about a medical problem, never hesitate to consult your doctor or another trained healthcare professional. Never ignore medical advice from professionals or put off getting it because of something you've read in this book.

The correctness, application, fitness, and completeness of the information in this book are not warranted or represented by the author or publisher. They make no representations regarding merchantability, fitness for a particular purpose, or implicit or stated guarantees. Never will the writer or publisher be held accountable for any kind of loss or other damages, including but not limited to special, incidental, consequential, or other damages.

The views and opinions expressed in this book are those of the author and do not necessarily reflect the official policy or position of any other individual, agency, organization, or company.

About the author

Winnie R. Adams, the author of "Optimizing Her Fertility: A Comprehensive Guide to Enhance Conception through Diet, Lifestyle, and Strategic Supplements," is a passionate advocate for reproductive health and wellness. With a background in Nutrition, Adams brings a unique blend of expertise, empathy, and a commitment to empowering individuals on their fertility journey.

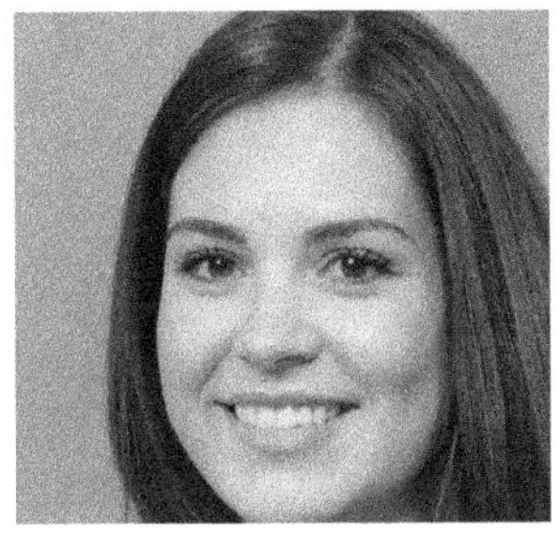

Having witnessed the challenges that many face in their quest for parenthood, Adams embarked on extensive research, delving into the realms of nutrition, lifestyle, and holistic approaches to fertility. This book is a culmination of not only scientific knowledge but also a heartfelt understanding of the emotional nuances that accompany the pursuit of a growing family.

Adams believes in the power of education and aims to demystify the complexities of fertility, providing readers with a comprehensive guide that goes beyond generic advice. The author's dedication to evidence-based information, coupled with a warm and relatable writing style, makes "Optimizing Her Fertility" a trustworthy companion for those navigating the often-intricate path to conception. In addition to her writing, Adams strives to foster a supportive community where individuals can find guidance, inspiration, and practical solutions on their fertility journey.

"Optimizing Her Fertility" is not just a book for Adams, but a shared journey with readers, a testament to the belief that everyone deserves the knowledge and tools to make informed choices about their reproductive health. As Adams invites you to explore the pages of this guide, she hopes to empower you with the insights and strategies needed to enhance your fertility and pave the way for the joy of parenthood.

TABLE OF CONTENT

INTRODUCTION

In the intricate tapestry of life, the desire to conceive and nurture a new beginning is a profound and universal aspiration. However, for many individuals and couples, the journey toward parenthood can be met with challenges and complexities, often leaving them in the uncharted territory of infertility. "Optimizing Her Fertility: A Comprehensive Guide to Enhance Conception through Diet, Lifestyle, and Strategic Supplements" seeks to be a beacon of hope and knowledge for those embarking on this transformative quest.

This book is not merely a compilation of facts and figures; it is a roadmap designed to empower individuals and couples with a deep understanding of infertility and, more importantly, the tools to overcome it. Our exploration begins with an in-depth analysis of the various facets of infertility, unraveling the mysteries behind conditions such as PCOS, hormonal imbalance, unexplained infertility, endometriosis, and blocked tubes. Each chapter delves into the symptoms, causes, diagnosis, and treatment options, ensuring that readers are equipped with comprehensive insights into their unique fertility challenges.

Navigating the landscape of fertility requires more than just medical knowledge—it demands a holistic approach. Recognizing this, we dedicate significant chapters to the pivotal role of nutrition in optimizing fertility. From breakfast choices to sumptuous main dishes, side dishes, and delectable desserts, our fertility diet principles are crafted to be inclusive, catering to the preferences of both vegetarians and non-vegetarians. The recipes provided are not only nourishing but also designed to support reproductive health, creating a harmonious balance between taste and fertility-friendly ingredients.

Beyond dietary considerations, this guide explores therapeutic interventions and the strategic use of supplements. Emphasizing a comprehensive and integrative approach, we aim to empower readers to take charge of their fertility journey, collaborating with healthcare professionals while implementing practical lifestyle changes that can positively influence their reproductive well-being.

Embarking on the path to parenthood is a deeply personal and often challenging experience. "Optimizing Her Fertility" invites you to embark on this journey with knowledge, confidence, and a personalized plan tailored to your unique needs. May this book serve as a guiding light, illuminating the way toward the realization of your most cherished dreams—the creation of new life and the joy of parenthood.

Overview of Optimizing Her Fertility

Embarking on the journey to parenthood can be a deeply personal and sometimes challenging experience. "Optimizing Her Fertility" is your go-to companion, designed to demystify the complexities of infertility and empower you with a holistic approach to enhance your chances of conception.

Understanding Infertility:

We kick things off by diving into the nitty-gritty of infertility. Whether it's PCOS, hormonal imbalance, unexplained infertility, endometriosis, or blocked tubes, we unpack the symptoms, causes, and treatment options, providing you with a solid foundation to navigate your unique fertility challenges.

Fertility Diagnostics:

Knowledge is power, especially when it comes to fertility diagnostics. This chapter guides you through medical tests, helping you decipher results and collaborate effectively with healthcare professionals to make informed decisions about your fertility journey.

Fertility Diet Magic:

As the popular saying goes" We are what we eat". We not only outline the principles of a fertility-friendly diet but also serve up delicious recipes for breakfast, soups, salads, main dishes, side dishes, and desserts. And don't worry, whether you're a vegetarian or a meat lover, we've got you covered.

Therapies and Supplements:

Taking a holistic approach, we explore therapies and supplements that complement your dietary efforts. From lifestyle changes to strategic supplement use, this chapter is your guide to practical interventions to boost fertility.

The Path Forward:

As we wrap up, we synthesize the key takeaways and encourage you to chart your personalized path forward. Armed with newfound knowledge and understanding, you'll be ready to navigate your fertility journey with confidence.

 Optimizing Her Fertility" isn't just a book; it's a friend on your fertility journey, offering a blend of science, practical advice, and mouth-watering recipes to inspire and support you on your path to parenthood. Let's embark on this transformative journey

CHAPTER 1: UNDERSTANDING INFERTILITY

Infertility is diagnosed when a woman has tried to conceive for more than six months (Age 35 and above) or over a year (Below 35) without conception. Trying to conceive here emphasizes having regular unprotected intercourse at least three days a week and during the ovulation period. In this chapter, we are going to give insight into five popular causes of infertility.

1. **PCOS (Polycystic Ovarian Syndrome)**: Symptoms, Causes, Diagnosis, Treatment

Symptoms: PCOS (Polycystic Ovarian Syndrome), Women with PCOS might deal with irregular periods, ovarian cysts, unexpected weight gain, acne, multiple chain-like tiny cysts on one or both ovaries, and more body hair than usual.

Causes: PCOS is often tied to things like insulin resistance, imbalance in hormone levels, and even family history.

Diagnosis: Doctors usually figure this out through a chat about your health, a physical exam, a Transvaginal or Pelvic ultrasound, and some blood tests to check hormones.

Treatment: Managing PCOS often involves lifestyle tweaks like a balanced diet and exercise, along with medications to help regulate periods and tackle symptoms.

2. **Hormonal Imbalance**: Unraveling the Complexities

Hormonal imbalances can mess with your reproductive system, your metabolism, and even your mood.

Causes can range from stress, aging, and medical conditions to lifestyle choices.

Diagnosing involves some blood tests to check how your hormones are doing, some of these hormones checked are FSH(Follicle Stimulating Hormone), LH(Luteinizing Hormone), Prolactin, Progesterone, Estrogen, Thyroid Hormones(T3, T4), Cortisol, etc.
Treatment might include hormone therapy, lifestyle changes, and tackling any underlying health issues.

3. **Unexplained Infertility**: Navigating the Unknown

Imagine trying to get pregnant, but there's no clear reason why it's not happening, that's unexplained infertility. Though if you ask me, I would say that there's always a reason hence it can be explained.

Causes: It could be small things like egg quality, sperm issues, or problems with implantation.

Diagnosis: Doctors figure this out by eliminating other known causes.

Treatment: Treatment may involve assisted reproductive technologies or making some lifestyle changes.

4. **Endometriosis**: A Deep Dive into Causes and Solutions

Causes: This occurs when tissue that resembles the uterus lining grows elsewhere in the body. This tissue may develop on the fallopian tubes, ovaries or bladder.

Symptoms: Serious pelvic pain, heavy periods, and trouble getting pregnant.

Diagnosis: They often need to peek inside with surgery to be sure, this procedure is known as Laparoscopy.

Solutions: Managing endometriosis could mean dealing with pain, hormones, or even surgery, depending on how severe it is.

5. **Blocked Tubes**: Identifying and Addressing Obstructions

Causes: Tubes get blocked due to things like infections, scar tissue, or past inflammation.

Symptoms: You might struggle to get pregnant, feel pelvic pain, or notice irregular periods.

Diagnosis: Special tests like HSG or laparoscopy can spot these blockages.

Addressing Obstructions: Fixing blockages might involve surgery, fertility drugs, or methods like IVF, depending on how serious it is.

CHAPTER 2: FERTILITY DIAGNOSTICS

Navigating the landscape of fertility can feel like deciphering a complex puzzle, where every piece matters, it can be frustrating and unending. In this journey, the role of medical tests and evaluations becomes a crucial guidepost, illuminating the path toward understanding and ultimately enhancing fertility.

The Role of Medical Tests and Evaluations in Fertility:

Embarking on the quest for parenthood often involves a series of diagnostic tests that serve as a roadmap to uncover potential barriers to conception. These tests are designed to scrutinize various aspects of reproductive health, from hormonal balance and ovarian function to sperm quality. As much as these tests may feel like a maze, they are invaluable tools in providing insights into the intricacies of fertility.

Interpreting Diagnostic Results:

Once the tests are complete, the next challenge arises: interpreting the results. It's like unraveling a story encoded in numbers and charts. This is where collaboration with knowledgeable healthcare professionals becomes pivotal. Understanding what these results mean for your fertility journey can be empowering, it offers clarity on potential hurdles and guides the formulation of a personalized plan.

Collaborating with Healthcare Professionals:

Embarking on the fertility journey is not a solitary endeavor. Collaborating with healthcare professionals becomes a partnership, a shared commitment to unraveling the complexities and optimizing reproductive health. Open communication is key, creating a space where questions are welcomed, and concerns are addressed. A collaborative approach ensures that the expertise of healthcare professionals aligns with the unique nuances of an individual's fertility challenges.

In this collaborative process, healthcare professionals become allies, providing not just medical expertise but also emotional support. Navigating the emotional roller coaster of fertility challenges can be daunting, and having a healthcare team that understands both the science and the emotions involved is invaluable.

As the results of medical tests shape the narrative of your fertility journey, remember that they are not verdicts but rather compass points guiding the way forward. They empower you with knowledge, enabling you to make informed decisions about potential treatments, lifestyle adjustments, or assisted reproductive technologies.

In essence, the role of medical tests and evaluations in fertility is more than just data collection.It's a testament to the strides we've made in reproductive medicine, providing hope and actionable insights for those who dream of creating new life. Remember, in this journey, every test, every result, and every collaboration is a step forward – a step closer to the fulfillment of the timeless dream of parenthood.

List of Tests to diagnose Fertility Challenges

In the realm of reproductive health, the onset of infertility can be an emotionally challenging experience for women and their partners. Female infertility refers to the inability of a woman to conceive within a given timeframe, typically after regular, unprotected sexual intercourse for one year. Ignited by a plethora of potential factors, such as hormonal imbalances and structural abnormalities, female infertility serves as a complex and multifaceted issue that necessitates a comprehensive diagnostic approach. The purpose of this chapter is to outline and discuss the essential tests that should be conducted to identify and diagnose the underlying causes of female infertility. By understanding the various diagnostic methods available, medical professionals can effectively assess, treat, and provide support to individuals facing these challenges. Through an in-depth exploration of these diagnostic procedures, this chapter aims to shed light on the complexity of female infertility and highlight the importance of tailored diagnostic approaches to enhance patient care.

Hormonal Tests

Hormonal tests play a crucial role in diagnosing female infertility. These tests help to assess the levels of various hormones in the body, which can provide valuable insights into ovulation patterns, hormonal imbalances, and reproductive health. One essential test is the measurement of follicle-stimulating hormone (FSH) levels. FSH stimulates the growth and development of follicles in the ovaries, and abnormal levels can indicate issues with ovarian function. Another important hormone to evaluate is luteinizing hormone (LH). LH triggers ovulation and high levels can indicate problems with ovulation. Additionally, measuring levels of estradiol, progesterone, and thyroid-stimulating hormone (TSH) can provide further information about ovarian function and hormonal imbalances that may be contributing to infertility. These hormonal tests, along with a comprehensive evaluation of other factors, enable healthcare professionals to accurately diagnose and treat female infertility.

Ovulation Tests

Ovulation tests are an essential tool used in diagnosing female infertility. These tests are designed to detect the surge in luteinizing hormone (LH) that occurs just before ovulation. By measuring the LH levels in the urine or blood, ovulation tests can accurately predict the fertile window of a woman's menstrual cycle. This information is crucial for couples who are trying to conceive as it helps them time intercourse for optimal chances of pregnancy. Ovulation tests are available in various formats, including urine-based test strips, midstream tests, and digital ovulation monitors. Studies have shown that ovulation tests are reliable and effective in identifying the fertile period. However, it is important to note that they do not confirm ovulation itself, but rather the impending release of an egg. Thus, additional tests and evaluations may be necessary to determine the cause of infertility if ovulation tests indicate normal results.

Imaging Tests

Imaging tests play a crucial role in the diagnosis of female infertility. These tests help identify any anatomical abnormalities or structural issues that may be affecting a woman's reproductive system. One commonly used imaging test is transvaginal ultrasound, which provides detailed images of the uterus, ovaries, and fallopian tubes. This test can help detect abnormalities such as uterine fibroids, ovarian cysts, or tubal blockages. Another imaging test that may be used is hysterosalpingography, which involves injecting a contrast dye into the uterus and taking X-ray images to visualize the shape and structure of the uterus and fallopian tubes. Magnetic resonance imaging (MRI) may also be employed in certain cases to provide more detailed images of the pelvic organs. These imaging tests, along with other diagnostic techniques, help healthcare professionals determine the underlying causes of infertility and devise appropriate treatment plans.

Genetic Tests

Genetic tests play a significant role in diagnosing female infertility. These tests evaluate the genetic makeup of individuals and identify any genetic mutations or abnormalities that could be causing infertility. One commonly used genetic test is karyotyping, which examines the structure and number of chromosomes in a person's cells. This test can detect chromosomal abnormalities such as Turner syndrome or variants in the X and Y chromosomes that may contribute to infertility. Another genetic test used to diagnose female infertility is the Fragile X syndrome test. Fragile X syndrome is the most common inherited cause of intellectual disability and can also affect fertility in women. A Fragile X syndrome test detects mutations in the Fragile X mental retardation 1 (FMR1) gene, which can help determine if the gene mutation is contributing to infertility. By identifying genetic factors that may be causing female infertility, these genetic tests provide essential information for developing personalized treatment plans to address infertility issues.

In conclusion, diagnosing female infertility requires a comprehensive approach that includes a multitude of tests and examinations. These tests can be categorized into different categories, including blood tests, imaging tests, and specialized procedures. Blood tests such as hormone level measurements provide crucial insights into the functioning of the reproductive system. Imaging tests like ultrasounds help visualize the reproductive organs and identify any abnormalities. Specialized procedures, such as hysterosalpingogram and laparoscopy, can further assess the health of the uterus and fallopian tubes. By conducting these tests systematically and analyzing the results comprehensively, healthcare professionals can accurately diagnose the causes of female infertility and develop appropriate treatment plans. Furthermore, ongoing research and advancements in medical technology are continually improving the diagnostic processes and expanding the range of available tests, offering hope for better outcomes in the future. Overall, a thorough understanding and implementation of these necessary tests are vital for effectively diagnosing female infertility.

CHAPTER 3 FERTILITY DIET PRINCIPLES

Infertility is a major problem in today's society and recurs in as much as 20–30% of the fertile female population. The World Health Organization (WHO) also reports that up to 80 million women world-wide have been affected by this disease to date, with a prevalence of 50% of all women in developing countries. Besides, several gynecological and systemic diseases affecting a woman's fertility, there are other factors too that contribute greatly to this problem such as unhealthy lifestyle, poor environmental conditions, Strenuous Jobs, poor and unbalanced diet all interfere with reproduction safety in both women and men.

How nutrition affects fertility

The body needs certain nutrients to function and these nutrients are not to be consumed in excess or less. Abnormal body weight, as well as dietary enrichment in carbohydrates, fatty acids, proteins, vitamins, and minerals all, exert a detrimental impact on both ovulatory function and normal spermatogenesis. Nutrients play an important role in female fertility because several nutrients of major diets also affect the implantation of a normal embryo.

It is necessary to have appropriate food and balanced nutrients for optimal performance of the reproductive system. An unbalanced caloric and protein intake due to inappropriate food consumption, responsible for severe under- or overweight, leads to alterations of the ovarian function with a subsequent increase in infertility. Variations of the body weight in terms of obesity and overweight associated with alterations of the energy balance are also suspected to produce ovulatory disorders. According to the Occupational Safety and Health Administration (OSHA), long-lasting exposure to chemical agents as organic solvents, heavy metals, aromatic amines, pesticides, and vegetal toxins is related to reduced fertility and improved predisposition to occasional or recurrent miscarriages.

Principles to enhance Fertility

1. Eat foods rich in antioxidants

Folate and zinc are good examples of antioxidants that may improve fertility for both men and women. They get rid of free radicals in the body, as presence of these radicals can damage both sperm and egg cells.

Another study of 232 women showed that higher folate intake was associated with higher rates of implantation, clinical pregnancy, and live birth.

Examples of foods that are rich in antioxidants include fruits, vegetables, nuts, and grains. They are packed full of beneficial antioxidants like vitamins C and E, folate and beta carotene.

More of these healthy foods should be incorporated into our daily diet.

2. Eat a bigger breakfast

Eating breakfast may help women with fertility problems. Studies show that rather than skipping breakfast, eating larger breakfast may improve fertility in women especially with PCOS

For moderate weight women with PCOS, eating most of their calories at breakfast reduced insulin levels by 8 percent and testosterone levels by 50 percent. High levels of either can contribute to infertility.

Eating larger breakfast and smaller dinner allowed women to ovulate more and better than women who ate a smaller breakfast and larger dinner, suggesting improved fertility.

However, one should be careful when increasing the size of your breakfast because it may likely lead to weight gain.

3. Avoid trans fats

Eating healthy fats every day is important for boosting fertility and overall health.Consuming trans fats have negative effects on insulin sensitivity and also affects ovulation in women.

Trans fats are commonly found in hydrogenated vegetable oils and are usually present in some margarine, fried foods, processed products, and baked goods.

Studies have found that a diet higher in trans fats and lower in unsaturated fats was linked to infertility for both men and women.

4. Eat Fewer carbs if you are diagnosed with PCOS

Eating a lower carb diet (where less than 45 percent of calories come from carbs) is generally recommended for women with PCOS.

Several studies have indicated that managing carb intake provides beneficial effects on some aspects of PCOS.

Low carb diets may help to maintain a healthy weight, stabilize insulin levels, and aid fat loss, it can also help regulate the menstrual cycle.

5. Eat fewer refined carbs

The type of Carb consumed has a great influence on fertility, complex carbs are more fertility friendly unlike refined carbs

Refined carbs may be especially problematic. Examples of refined carbs include sugary foods, carbonated drinks and processed grains, including white pasta, bread, and rice.

Refined carbs are absorbed very quickly into the blood causing spikes in blood sugar and insulin levels. They also have a high glycemic index (GI). Glycemic index indicates if a carbohydrate-dense food will raise your blood sugar significantly.

Insulin is chemically similar to ovarian hormones. These hormones help our eggs mature. Consistent high insulin levels affect the body's ability to produce reproductive hormones. This can interrupt ovulation and also affect egg quality.

Because PCOS is associated with high insulin levels, consuming refined carbs makes the symptoms even worse

6. Increase your fiber intake

Including more fiber in your diet helps your body eliminate excess hormones and maintains balanced blood sugar levels. Certain types of fiber can assist in removing excess estrogen from the body by binding to it in the intestines, leading to its elimination as waste. High-fiber foods like whole grains, fruits, vegetables, and beans can contribute to this. Women are recommended to consume 25 grams of fiber per day, while men should aim for 31 grams.

Studies have shown that higher cereal fiber intake is linked to a 44 percent lower risk of ovulatory infertility in women over 32. However, findings on fiber's impact are still mixed, as another study indicated that a 5-gram daily increase in fiber could decrease hormone concentration and increase the likelihood of anovulation.

To determine if you need to adjust your fiber intake, consult with your doctor.

7.Substitute animal proteins with plant-based alternatives

Reducing the intake of animal proteins, such as meat, fish, and eggs, in favor of plant-based sources like beans, nuts, and seeds, is associated with a reduced risk of infertility. Studies suggest that even a small shift of 5 percent of total calories from animal to vegetable protein can decrease the risk of ovulatory infertility by over 50 percent.

Consider incorporating more vegetable, bean, lentil, nut, and low-mercury fish proteins into your diet for a healthier balance.

8.Opt for high-fat dairy

Contrary to low-fat dairy, high-fat dairy consumption has been associated with a decreased risk of infertility. A comprehensive study in 2007 revealed that women who consumed one or more servings of high-fat dairy per day were 27 percent less likely to be infertile.

To potentially benefit from this, try replacing one daily serving of low-fat dairy with a high-fat alternative, like whole milk or full-fat yogurt.

9.Include a multivitamin in your routine

Taking multivitamins may reduce the likelihood of ovulatory infertility, as micronutrients in vitamins play essential roles in fertility. For those trying to conceive, a multivitamin containing folate may be particularly beneficial.

Discuss supplement options, including multivitamins, with your doctor to align them with your pregnancy goals.

10.Stay physically active in moderation

Moderate physical activity positively influences fertility for both men and women, especially for those with obesity. However, excessive high-intensity exercise can have the opposite effect, potentially disrupting hormonal balance and increasing stress hormones.

If planning to increase activity, do so gradually and inform your healthcare team. Incorporate slow-weighted exercises and some yoga poses, known to be beneficial for female fertility.

11.Manage stress levels

Increased stress levels can decrease the chances of pregnancy due to hormonal changes. While research on stress and fertility is mixed, receiving support and counseling can reduce anxiety and depression levels, enhancing the likelihood of conception.

Don't forget to take time for yourself to relax and unwind.

12.Limit caffeine intake

Although evidence on the link between caffeine and fertility is inconclusive, some studies suggest a potential delay in conception with high caffeine intake. To be cautious, consider limiting caffeine to one or two cups of coffee per day.

Explore non-coffee alternatives for a healthier choice.

13.Maintain a healthy weight

Weight plays a significant role in fertility for both men and women. Whether underweight or overweight, these conditions are associated with increased infertility due to their impact on menstrual function.

Collaborate with your healthcare provider to achieve a healthy and sustainable weight through tailored guidance.

14.Monitor iron levels

Consuming iron supplements and non-heme iron from plant-based sources may reduce the risk of ovulatory infertility. While more evidence is needed, it's advisable to check iron levels with your doctor and consider iron-rich foods along with vitamin C for enhanced absorption.

15.Keep alcohol in check

Consuming alcohol can have a negative impact on fertility, although the specific amount that may cause this effect remains uncertain.

A study indicated that having more than 14 alcoholic drinks per week was linked to a longer time taken to conceive. Another study involving 7,393 women discovered that a high alcohol intake was associated with an increased likelihood of undergoing infertility examinations.

However, the evidence regarding moderate alcohol consumption is conflicting. An older study found no connection between moderate drinking and infertility, while other studies suggest that moderate intake can influence fertility.

CHAPTER 4: NOURISHING BREAKFAST FOR FERTILITY

Embarking on a journey to enhance fertility begins with the very first meal of the day. In this chapter, we explore breakfast options that are rich in nutrients, crafted to kickstart your morning and promote reproductive health. From delightful smoothie bowls to hearty omelets, each recipe is thoughtfully designed with ingredients to boost fertility, aiming to nourish your body and set a positive tone for the day.

Breakfast Ideas for Fertility
1. Whole Milk Porridge with Blueberries and Chia Seeds
Kick off your day with a satisfying bowl of porridge, featuring oats known for their comforting warmth and long-lasting fullness. Opting for whole milk, as studies suggest, might offer more protective benefits compared to reduced-fat alternatives. For those following a vegan or plant-based diet, various plant milks can provide a nutritious and delicious alternative.
Enhance your porridge with chia seeds, tiny powerhouses of antioxidants, omega-3s, and fiber. Add a touch of sweetness and extra antioxidants with blueberries, along with some nuts or nut butter for a luxurious taste. These simple additions create a delicious and healthy breakfast, setting a positive tone for the day ahead.
Ingredients:

- Oats
- Whole milk e.g Almond milk
- 1 large handful of blueberries
- 1 Teaspoon of Chia seeds

Method:
Cook oats on low heat for one to three minutes.
Once ready drop and serve with milk, blueberries and chia seeds as toppings
Serve warm or cold.

2. Smoked Salmon and Scrambled Eggs on Whole Grain Toast

Boosting your omega-3 fatty acids is crucial for fertility, and incorporating oily fish like smoked salmon into your breakfast a few times a week is a delectable way to achieve this. Omega-3s not only support fetal development but are also linked to improved egg quality and extended reproductive lifespan. If fish isn't your preference, eggs are an excellent alternative. Eggs provide essential nutrients like choline, crucial for placental function and early brain development, along with B12, B6, vitamin D, selenium, zinc, iron, and amino acids necessary for growth and development.

Starting your day with smoked salmon and scrambled eggs on wholegrain toast can be a tasty and nutritious choice, benefiting both you and your future baby.

3. Green Vegetable Frittata

Boosting folate levels, essential for pregnancy, can be achieved by incorporating green leafy veggies like spinach, kale, and asparagus into your diet. Paired with eggs, these vegetables contribute to the ultimate fertility breakfast. Leafy greens not only provide fiber but also offer antioxidants, making them a valuable addition to a healthy diet. Using a muffin tray for a frittata batch allows for easy preparation and storage in the freezer, ensuring a convenient and nutrient-packed breakfast.

Ingredients for one large frittata:
- 1 teaspoon of olive oil
- 2 handfuls of your preferred leafy green vegetables
- 1 large handful of spinach
- ½ cup of chopped onions
- 2-3 free-range eggs
- Feta cheese or cheese of your choice
- Salt and pepper for seasoning

Method:
Preheat your oven to 180°C.
Sauté chopped veggies in a pan with olive oil until soft.
Add onions and cook for a few minutes.
Add spinach, season with salt and pepper.
Arrange vegetables in an oven-proof pan.

Beat eggs, pour over vegetables, and sprinkle cheese on top.
Bake for 20 minutes or until set and golden.
Serve warm or cold.

4. Whole Grain Granola with Full-Fat Greek Yogurt

For a healthy and delightful breakfast or snack, granola made from whole grains, nuts, seeds, and low-sugar recipes is an excellent choice. Packed with fertility-supporting nutrients like healthy fats, zinc, and antioxidants, a good granola can be fulfilling and satisfying. Opt for a low-sugar homemade granola paired with full-fat Greek yogurt, which not only enhances bone health with calcium but also supports a healthy gut bacterial balance with probiotics.

Granola Ingredients:
- 4 cups rolled oats
- 1 ½ cup raw nuts and/or seeds
- ½ teaspoon salt
- ½ teaspoon ground cinnamon
- ½ cup coconut oil or olive oil
- ½ cup maple syrup or honey
- 1 teaspoon vanilla extract
- ⅔ cup dried fruit

Granola Method:
Preheat the oven to 180°C
Combine oats, nuts/seeds, salt, and cinnamon in a bowl.

Add oil, maple syrup/honey, and vanilla, mixing until coated.

Spread on the prepared pan and bake for 20-25 minutes, stirring halfway.

Cool for 45 minutes, top with dried fruit, and break into pieces.

5. Black Beans and Avocado on Whole-Grain Toast

For a vegan-friendly fertility breakfast, consider black beans and avocado on whole-grain toast. Black beans, rich in vegetarian protein and fiber, align with studies suggesting plant protein positively impacts fertility. Beans also contribute to folate intake, crucial for both expecting mothers and egg quality. Avocado, with its monounsaturated healthy fats, supports overall health and recent studies indicate potential improvements in women's fertility with an intake of these healthy fats over saturated fats. This nutrient-packed breakfast offers benefits for both general health and fertility.

6.Quinoa and Vegetable Stir-Fry:

- Ingredients: Quinoa, assorted vegetables (bell peppers, broccoli, carrots, peas), tofu or chicken, soy sauce, ginger, garlic.
- Instructions: Cook quinoa. In a pan, stir-fry tofu or chicken with veggies, ginger, and garlic. Add

cooked quinoa and soy sauce to stir-fry mixture. Toss until well combined.

7. Salmon and Sweet Potato Skewers:

- Ingredients: Salmon filets, sweet potatoes, olive oil, lemon, herbs (rosemary or thyme), salt, and pepper.
- Instructions: Cut salmon and sweet potatoes into chunks. Thread onto skewers. Brush with olive oil, lemon juice, and herbs. Grill until salmon is cooked through and sweet potatoes are tender.

8. Chickpea and Spinach Curry:

- Ingredients: Chickpeas, spinach, tomatoes, onions, garlic, ginger, curry spices (turmeric, cumin, coriander), coconut milk.
- Instructions: Sauté onions, garlic, and ginger. Add tomatoes and spices. Stir in chickpeas and spinach. Simmer until flavors meld. Finish with coconut milk.

9. Vegetarian Lentil Bolognese:

- Ingredients: Lentils, tomatoes, onions, carrots, garlic, tomato sauce, Italian herbs, whole wheat or gluten-free pasta.
- Instructions: Sauté onions, carrots, and garlic. Add cooked lentils, tomatoes, tomato sauce, and herbs. Simmer until it thickens. Serve over cooked pasta.

10.Grilled Chicken or Tofu Salad:
- Ingredients: Grilled chicken or tofu, mixed greens, cherry tomatoes, cucumber, feta cheese, balsamic vinaigrette.
- Instructions: Grill chicken or tofu. Assemble a salad with mixed greens, tomatoes, cucumber, and feta. Top with grilled protein and drizzle with balsamic vinaigrette.

11.Egg and Vegetable Fried Rice:
- Ingredients: Brown rice, eggs, mixed vegetables (peas, carrots, corn), soy sauce, sesame oil, ginger, garlic.
- Instructions: Cook brown rice. In a pan fry some scrambled eggs. Add mixed vegetables, ginger, and garlic. Stir in cooked rice, soy sauce, and a dash of sesame oil.

12 .Mushroom and Spinach Stuffed Bell Peppers:
- Ingredients: Bell peppers, mushrooms, spinach, quinoa, feta cheese (optional), Italian herbs.
- Instructions: Cut bell peppers in half. Sauté mushrooms and spinach. Mix with cooked quinoa and herbs. Stuff bell peppers, top with feta, and bake until peppers are tender.

CHAPTER 5: SOUPS AND SALADS FOR FERTILITY

Creating Culinary Delights: Infusing Fertility-Friendly Elements

In this chapter, let's explore the world of soups and salads, where flavors and nutrients come together to support fertility. Revel in the joy of crafting delectable and nutrient-rich soup and salad recipes that not only excite your taste buds but also contribute to your reproductive well-being. These recipes are carefully designed, ensuring that each spoonful or forkful aligns with your fertility aspirations.

Fertility-Boosting Soup Recipes

1. Anti-Inflammatory Fertility Soup

Ingredients:

- 3 Carrots, chopped
- 4 Celery Stalks, chopped
- 6 Garlic cloves, diced
- 1 Onion, medium size, chopped
- 1 Sweet potato, peeled and cubed
- 1 inch piece of ginger, peeled and chopped/grated
- 1 inch piece of turmeric, peeled and chopped/grated

- 1 can of diced tomatoes
- 4 cups of vegetable/chicken broth
- 1 cup of red lentils
- 2 cups of kale/spinach (frozen or fresh)
- 1 bunch of parsley
- 1 lemon
- Salt, pepper, and preferred spices
- Optional treat: Feta cheese

Bone Broth Soup for Fertility

Bone Broth Recipe:

- 2 lbs. of bones (cooked or raw), preferably beef, chicken, turkey wings, lamb, and beef tail
- 1 Medium Vidalia Onion or Sweet Onion, diced
- 2-4 cloves of whole garlic cloves (crushed, whole, or without skin)
- 1 tsp of turmeric or shave about 1 Tbl of fresh turmeric root
- 1 lemon cut into slices OR 1/4 cup of Raw Unfiltered Apple Cider Vinegar (or both)

Herb and Veggie Options:

- 1 or 2 Tbsp of basil, oregano, parsley – dried (or one bunch of each if fresh)
- 1 or 2 Tsp of thyme, rosemary
- 1/4 to 1/2 Tsp of cayenne pepper (optional, based on preference)

Basic Preparation:

Place all ingredients into a large stock pot or crockpot.

Use the best water available, prioritizing medicinal benefits over taste.

Bring to a boil, then immediately simmer for a minimum of 2 hours, or overnight if preferred.

After cooling to room temperature, skim off some fat solids if desired.

Remove veggies and bones via colander, pressing down to extract maximum flavor.

Store the broth in the refrigerator or freezer.

Importance of Bone Broth for Fertility

Bone broth offers trace amounts of essential nutrients like protein, calcium, iron, magnesium, sodium, zinc, potassium, and collagen. When combined with veggies, it extracts higher amounts of each nutrient.

1. Magnesium:

Balances fertility hormones, decreasing inflammation to improve implantation chances.

2. Calcium:

Alkalizes the body, promoting a healthier environment for conception by reducing uterine acidity. Essential for sperm production in men.

3. Potassium:

Crucial for both male and female reproductive health. Protects sperm in the highly acidic female reproductive environment and reduces ovarian cyst formation.

4. Hormone Regulation:

Easy to digest, bone broth provides gut healing properties that balance hormones and alleviate digestive issues, indirectly boosting fertility.

5. Boosts the Immune System:

Acts as a traditional remedy for cold and flu symptoms, fortifying the immune system against pathogens and strengthening gut lining.

6. Heals the Gut Lining:

Repairs gut lining with gelatin content, reducing inflammation and addressing conditions like "leaky gut," IBS, and Crohn's disease.

7. Blood Sugar Regulation:

Contains glycine, impacting insulin secretion, lowering blood sugar, and maintaining insulin sensitivity crucial for fertility.

By incorporating these nutrient-rich soups and salads into your diet, you not only savor delightful meals but also nourish your body for optimal fertility. Explore the benefits of each ingredient, understanding their impact on hormonal balance, immune support, gut health, and blood sugar regulation. As you embark on this fertility-friendly culinary journey, relish in the joy of fostering reproductive well-being through wholesome and flavorful recipes.

Fertility-Boosting Salad Recipe

Ingredients:

- 2 cups rinsed and chopped Organic Romaine Lettuce (or substitute with butterhead, green-leaf, or red-leaf lettuce)
- 1 cup chopped or sliced roasted chicken (or substitute with black beans, fried eggs, turkey muffins)
- 1 whole small/medium avocado, sliced or diced
- 1 sheet sliced organic Nori or other seaweed (certified Kosher for those with shellfish allergies)
- 1 tbsp Goji berries
- 10 organic olives (kalamata or black)
- Sprinkling of seeds based on your menstrual cycle phase (Pumpkin for pre-ovulatory, sesame or sunflower for luteal phase)
- Nuts if desired, like a handful of walnuts (around 16 pieces)

Dressing:

- 1 Tbsp Organic Extra Virgin Olive Oil
- 1 Tbsp Organic Apple Cider Vinegar (Bragg's is a good choice)
- Sprinkle of fresh ground pepper and sea salt

CHAPTER 6: DESSERTS FOR FERTILITY

Sweet Delights with Purpose: Gratifying Your Sweet Tooth

Who says desserts can't be fertility-friendly? In this chapter, we present dessert recipes that not only satisfy your sweet tooth but also align with your reproductive health goals. Suitable for both vegetarians and non-vegetarians, these delectable treats prove that you can indulge in the pleasure of desserts while staying mindful of your fertility journey.

Berry Bliss Smoothie Bowl:
- Bursting with antioxidants from berries, this smoothie bowl not only pleases your taste buds but also provides essential nutrients for fertility.

Dark Chocolate Avocado Mousse:
- Creamy and indulgent, this dessert combines the richness of dark chocolate with the fertility-boosting properties of avocados, high in healthy fats.

Almond and Berry Parfait:
- Layered with almond yogurt, fresh berries, and a sprinkle of almonds, this parfait is a delightful combination of flavors and fertility-friendly ingredients.

Chia Seed Pudding with Mango:

- Chia seeds, rich in omega-3 fatty acids, paired with the sweetness of mango, create a delicious and nutritious pudding.

Greek Yogurt with Honey and Walnuts:

- Greek yogurt, a great source of protein and probiotics, drizzled with honey and topped with walnuts for a fertility-friendly dessert.

Oatmeal Raisin Cookies:

- Sweetened with natural sugars and enriched with oats, these cookies offer a wholesome treat while avoiding refined sugars that may impact fertility.

Peach and Almond Crumble:

- Fresh peaches combined with a nutty almond crumble create a delightful dessert that is not only tasty but also incorporates fertility-friendly ingredients.

Coconut Bliss Balls:

- Made with coconut, nuts, and a touch of sweetness, these bliss balls are a convenient and tasty way to enjoy a fertility-friendly treat.

Banana Walnut Muffins:

- Bananas, rich in potassium and other nutrients, combined with the goodness of walnuts in a muffin for a delicious and fertility-conscious dessert.

Berry and Yogurt Popsicles:

- Blend mixed berries with yogurt, freeze into popsicles for refreshing treats with a burst of antioxidants and probiotics.

Remember, moderation and a balanced diet are key. These desserts can be enjoyed as part of an overall fertility-friendly meal plan, supporting your reproductive health goals.

CHAPTER 7: NATURAL THERAPIES

Embarking on the journey to optimal fertility extends beyond dietary choices. This chapter serves as a roadmap to a holistic approach, shedding light on therapies and lifestyle adjustments that can significantly enhance your fertility. We'll also delve into the strategic use of supplements to complement your efforts. Let's explore three major therapies that can make a profound difference.

Exercise: A Path to Fertility Wellness

Exercise is more than a routine; it's a powerful ally in enhancing female fertility. Here, we uncover the benefits of incorporating fertility-friendly workouts into your lifestyle.

Benefits of Exercise on Female Fertility:

Regulating Hormones:
- Regular exercise contributes to hormonal balance, ensuring optimal menstrual cycles and reproductive hormone levels like estrogen and progesterone.

Enhancing Blood Flow:
- Improved circulation, a byproduct of exercise, nourishes reproductive organs, promoting the health of ovaries and uterus.

Managing Stress Levels:

- Exercise acts as a natural stress-buster, reducing cortisol levels and creating a conducive environment for conception.

Balancing Weight:

- Maintaining a healthy weight is crucial for fertility, and exercise aids in weight management, preventing both underweight and overweight scenarios.

Boosting Ovulation:

- For women with irregular ovulation, exercise plays a pivotal role in restoring regular cycles and promoting the release of eggs.

Improving Insulin Sensitivity:

- Exercise addresses insulin resistance, particularly beneficial for conditions like polycystic ovary syndrome (PCOS).

Fertility-Friendly Exercises:

Cardiovascular Workouts:

- Engage in moderate aerobic exercises such as brisk walking, jogging, or cycling for at least 180 minutes per week.

Strength Training:

- Include resistance training exercises 2-3 times per week, focusing on major muscle groups.

Yoga:

- Gentle and restorative, yoga enhances flexibility and mindfulness. Incorporate yoga sessions into your routine.

Pilates:

- Improve core strength and posture with Pilates exercises, providing effective yet low-impact support for fertility.

Swimming:

- A full-body workout, swimming offers gentle yet impactful cardiovascular benefits. Regular sessions can boost overall fitness.

Frequency and Consistency:

- Cardiovascular Exercise: Aim for at least 150 minutes per week in moderate-intensity sessions.
- Strength Training: Include exercises 2-3 times weekly targeting major muscle groups.
- Yoga and Pilates: Incorporate 2-3 sessions per week for flexibility, relaxation, and core strength.
- Consistency is Key: Regularity is crucial; choose activities you enjoy to make exercise a sustainable part of your lifestyle.

Remember, consult a healthcare professional before starting a new exercise regimen, especially if you have underlying health conditions. The fertility journey is unique for each woman, and a holistic approach including exercise can be a positive and empowering step.

Castor Oil Pack Therapy: Nurturing Reproductive Wellness

For centuries, castor oil therapy has been a cornerstone in promoting healing, specifically within the reproductive system. Castor oil packs offer a unique contribution to women's health, fertility, and addressing conditions such as scar tissue, adhesions, fibroids, ovarian cysts, and blocked fallopian tubes.

How Castor Oil Packs Improve Fertility

Increases Circulation:
- Stimulates the circulatory system, facilitating fresh oxygenated blood flow to nourish reproductive organs.

Boosts Immune System Function:
- Enhances lymphatic movement, part of the body's immune system, to remove toxins and cleanse reproductive organs.

Promotes Detoxification:
- Increases circulation to the liver, supporting detoxification and improving liver function crucial for hormonal balance.

Reduces Inflammation & Pain:

- Combats inflammation and pain associated with various fertility issues, providing natural support alongside acupuncture.

Relieves Stress:

- Offers a therapeutic break, aiding stress relief by encouraging moments of self-care and rest.

How to Apply a Castor Oil Pack

Saturate a piece of cotton flannel:

- Use cold-pressed, pure castor oil.

Place it on the lower abdomen:

- Directly on the skin, covering the lower abdomen.

Cover with plastic wrap:

- Add a gentle heat source on top, like a hot water bottle or heating pad.

Rest for 30-60 minutes:

- Lie down and relax during the application.

Stay hydrated:

- Drink plenty of room-temperature water during and after the session.

How often to apply castor oil packs

- Apply at least 3-4 times a week for an hour, excluding the post-ovulation period if trying to conceive.

- During an IVF cycle, avoid using castor oil packs during the stimulation phase.
- If not trying to conceive, apply daily for 15-20 minutes.

Massage to Enhance Benefits:

- After each castor oil therapy session, massage the abdomen for 15-20 minutes in circular motions using coconut or olive oil.

Incorporating castor oil packs into your fertility journey provides a natural and holistic approach to women's health and reproductive wellness.

Massages: A Touch of Comfort and Wellness

To complement the benefits of exercise and castor oil therapy, massages offer an additional layer of support. After each castor oil therapy session, a 15-20 minute massage on the abdomen using coconut or olive oil can further enhance the therapeutic impact.

By embracing these holistic approaches to fertility, you empower yourself to nurture overall well-being, making strides toward optimizing your chances of conception. Always consult with healthcare professionals for personalized advice, understanding that the journey to fertility is unique for each woman.

CHAPTER 8: SUPPLEMENTS

In this chapter, we will delve into the strategic use of supplements to complement your efforts. Some of these supplements we will be talking about include:

- Coenzyme Q10 (CoQ10):

Benefits: CoQ10 is an antioxidant that supports cellular energy production and may enhance egg and sperm health.

Dosage: Generally, a dosage of 100-200 mg per day is commonly recommended for fertility support.

- L-Arginine:

Benefits: L-Arginine is an amino acid that may improve blood flow to the reproductive organs, supporting overall fertility.

Dosage: Dosages often range from 1,000 to 3,000 mg per day, but individual needs may vary.

- Maca Root:

Benefits: Maca may help balance hormones and improve fertility, especially in women.

Dosage: Typical dosage ranges from 1,500 to 3,000 mg per day.

- Omega-3 Fish Oil (EPA and DHA):

Benefits: Omega-3 fatty acids support overall reproductive health, including regulating hormones and reducing inflammation.

Dosage: Aim for 1,000-2,000 mg of combined EPA and DHA per day.

- Chromium:

Benefits: Chromium is involved in insulin regulation, which may be beneficial for women with PCOS or insulin resistance affecting fertility.

Dosage: A common dosage is around 200-400 mcg per day.

- Inositol:

Benefits: Inositol, especially myo-inositol, may improve insulin sensitivity and support regular ovulation in women with PCOS.

Dosage: A typical dose ranges from 2,000 to 4,000 mg per day.

- DIM (Diindolylmethane):

Benefits: DIM supports estrogen metabolism, promoting a balance between estrogen and progesterone.

Dosage: Dosages typically range from 100 to 200 mg per day.

- Berberine:

Benefits: Berberine may help manage insulin resistance and improve fertility, particularly in women with PCOS.

Dosage: Commonly, 500-1,500 mg per day is recommended.

- N-Acetyl Cysteine (NAC):

Benefits: NAC is an antioxidant that may improve egg quality and reduce inflammation, supporting fertility.

Dosage: A common dosage is around 600-1,800 mg per day.

- Turmeric and Curcumin:

Benefits: Turmeric's anti-inflammatory properties, primarily due to curcumin, may support reproductive health.

Dosage: While turmeric can be included in the diet, curcumin supplements typically range from 500 to 2,000 mg per day.

Always consult with a healthcare professional before adding new supplements to your routine, especially if you are pregnant, breastfeeding, or taking other medications. Dosages may vary based on individual health conditions and specific fertility goals.

BONUS PAGE- Green juices and Smoothie recipes

Fertility Juice Recipes

Recipe 1   Ingredient

- 1 green apple

- 3 stalks of celery

- a handful of spinach

- 1 piece of ginger

Directions:

Add all ingredients in a juice extractor and extract the juice into a glass and drink either chilled or at room temperature; if using a blender, add all ingredients into a blender and blend until smooth then sieve to extract your juice to drink either chilled or at room temperature.

Recipe 2   Ingredient

- 1 big cucumber

- small bunch of kale leaves

- 1 green apple, 4 carrots

- quarter of broccoli

- quarter cabbage

Recipe 3   Ingredient

- 5 carrots

- 1-piece ginger
- 1 fresh tomato
- 1 green apple
- 2 beetroot

Recipe 4   Ingredient

- 4 tomatoes
- 2 carrots
- A small bunch parsley
- Half of small onion
- 1 cucumber
- 1 red pepper
- 1 clove of garlic and
- A small bunch of parsley

Recipe 5   Ingredients

- 3 strawberries
- Small Swiss charge
- A small bunch of kale leaves
- A handful of spinach

Recipe 6   Ingredients

- 2 beetroot

- 2 asparagus
- 1-piece ginger
- 4 carrots
- 1 large green apple
- Half cucumber
- Handful spinach leaves

Recipe 7   Ingredients

- Half cabbage
- Quarter cauliflower
- 1 English pear
- 2 stalks of Celery
- 1 clove of garlic
- 1 piece of garlic and
- 1 red pepper

Recipe 8   Ingredients

- Half broccoli head and stem
- 1 piece of ginger
- 1 piece of turmeric
- 2 English pears
- 1 cucumber

- Dandelion leaves
- 4 carrots and
- small bunch of cilantros

Recipe 9   Ingredients

- 6 carrots
- 2 tomatoes
- 2 beetroot
- 4 strawberries
- 1 ginger
- 1 turmeric
- A handful of spinach

Recipe 10 Ingredients

- Quarter cabbage
- Quarter cauliflower
- Quarter arugula leaves
- Small bunch of kale leaves
- Quarter of broccoli head and stem

Fertility Smoothie Recipes

Recipe 1   Ingredients

- ½ fresh peach or ½ cup of frozen peaches

- Quarter tablespoon ground cinnamon

- 1 tablespoon hemp seed

- 1 tablespoon chia seed (soaked in a little water for 2 hours)

- 1 teaspoon spirulina powder

- ½ cup coconut or almond milk

- Ice if using fresh peaches

Directions: Add all ingredients into the blender and blend until smooth and empty into a glass cup and enjoy. Remember: smoothies must not be stored, you make them and take within 15 mins

Recipe 2   Ingredients

- Quarter red grapefruit

- Quarter fresh/frozen strawberries

- ½ cup coconut milk

- ½ teaspoon vanilla extract

- 2 tablespoon peanut butter

- Add little water to make it less thick to your desire.

Recipe 3   Ingredients

- ½ tablespoon almond butter

- ½ teaspoon cinnamon powder

- 1 tablespoon flax seeds

- A little honey to taste

- 1 avocado

- 5-6 ice cubes (optional)

- Add little water to make it less thick

Recipe 4   Chia Pudding Smoothie Recipe

Ingredients

- 1 cup almond milk

- Half cup coconut milk

- 4 tablespoons of chia seed

- 2 tablespoons of honey

- Quarter teaspoon of cinnamon

- 1 scoop cocoa powder

- A handful coconut flakes

Recipe 5   Ingredients

- 1 avocado

- A handful spinach

- 1 tablespoon chia seed

- 1 tablespoon hemp seed

- A little honey to taste

- Add little water to make it less thick

Recipe 6   Ingredients

- ½ avocado

- 1 tablespoon cocoa powder

- 1 tablespoon spirulina powder

- 1 tablespoon soaked chia seeds

- ½ cup almond milk to serve as water

Recipe 7   Pineapple Core Implantation Smoothie Recipe (to be taken a day after ovulation for 5 days straight)

2 pieces of pineapple core

3 strawberries

4 blueberries

Half cup full fat yogurts

A handful spinach

CONCLUSION

Congratulations on reaching the end of "Optimizing Her Fertility"! As you close the final chapter of this book, take a moment to reflect on the incredible journey you've embarked upon towards parenthood.

Throughout these pages, we've explored the myriad ways in which diet, lifestyle, and strategic supplements can profoundly impact your fertility journey. From understanding the intricate connection between nutrition and reproductive health to implementing practical lifestyle changes, you've gained invaluable insights that will serve as your compass on this path.

But remember, the journey to parenthood is not always straightforward. It's okay to encounter setbacks, to feel overwhelmed, or to need support along the way. You are not alone. "Optimizing Her Fertility" is not just a book; it's a community of individuals, like you, who are dedicated to realizing their dreams of starting a family.

As you move forward, know that every step you take, every choice you make, brings you closer to your goal. Embrace the journey, celebrate the victories – big and small – and never lose sight of the hope and resilience that fuel your determination.

Above all, don't be hard on yourself. Keep doing the best you can, there's light at the end of the tunnel.

With "Optimizing Her Fertility" as your guide, may you continue to navigate this path with courage, optimism, and unwavering determination. Here's to new beginnings, to miracles in the making, and to the beautiful journey of parenthood that lies ahead.

Wishing you all the love, joy, and success on your fertility journey.